More Than Just Two

a celebration of egg donation

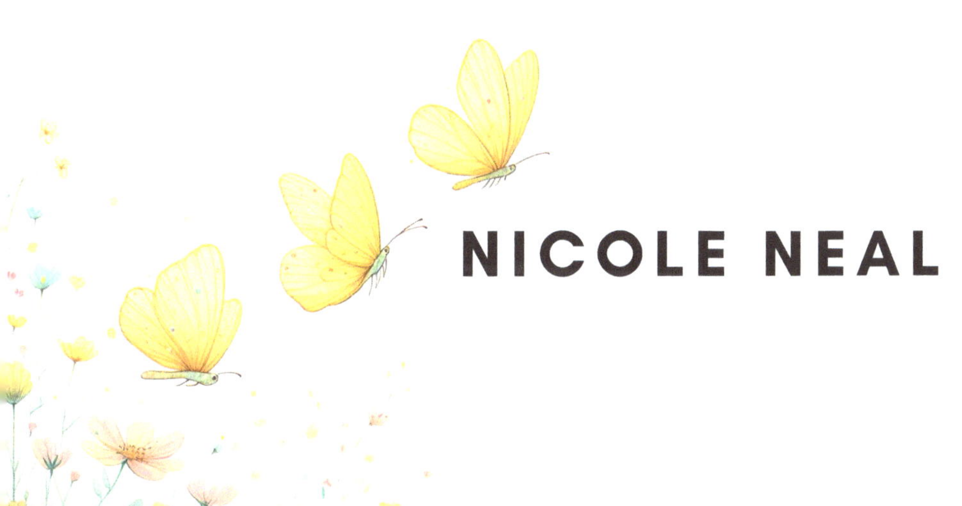

NICOLE NEAL

For my baby girl, her daddy, her egg donor,
and every speck of earthly dust,
all of which helped make me a mom.

When the rain feeds the seed
to grow into a tree,
the rich earth below
keeps it tall, strong, and steady.

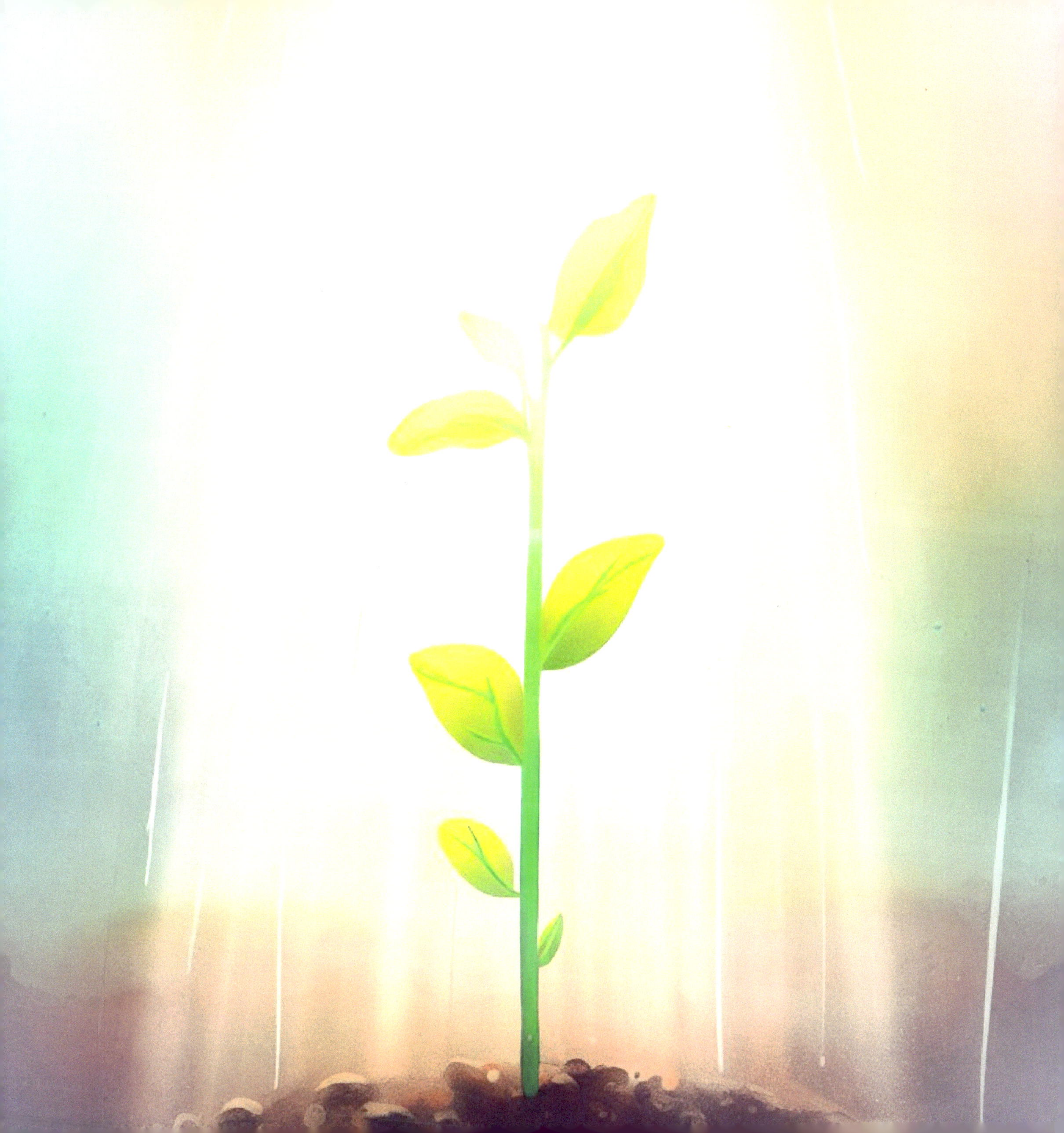

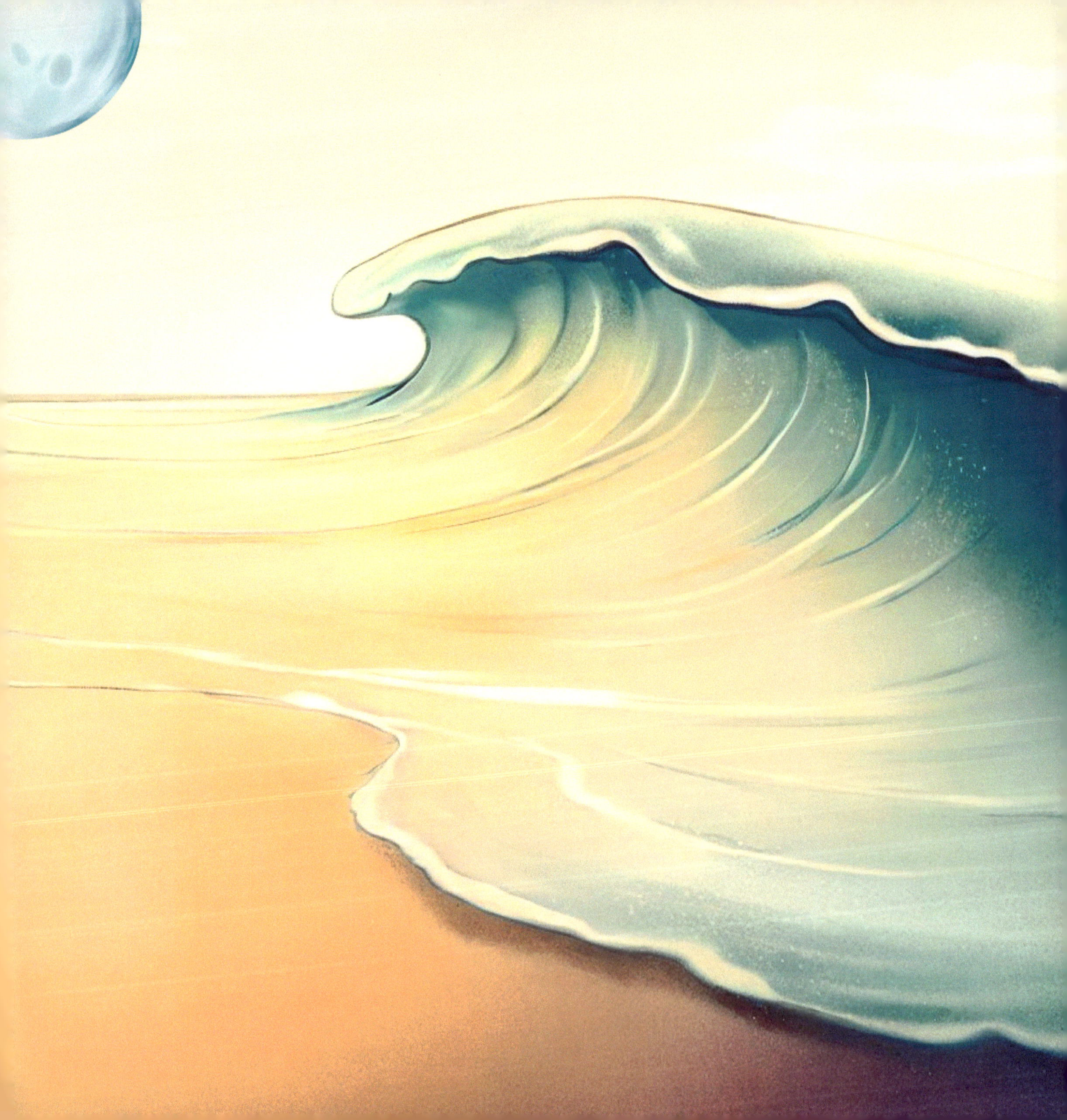

When the moon tugs on the ocean,

setting waves into motion,

the golden warm sand

is a soft place to land.

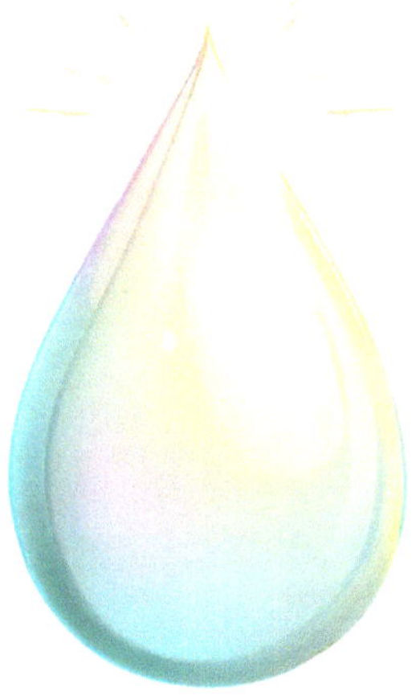

When the sunshine and water drops

perfectly align,

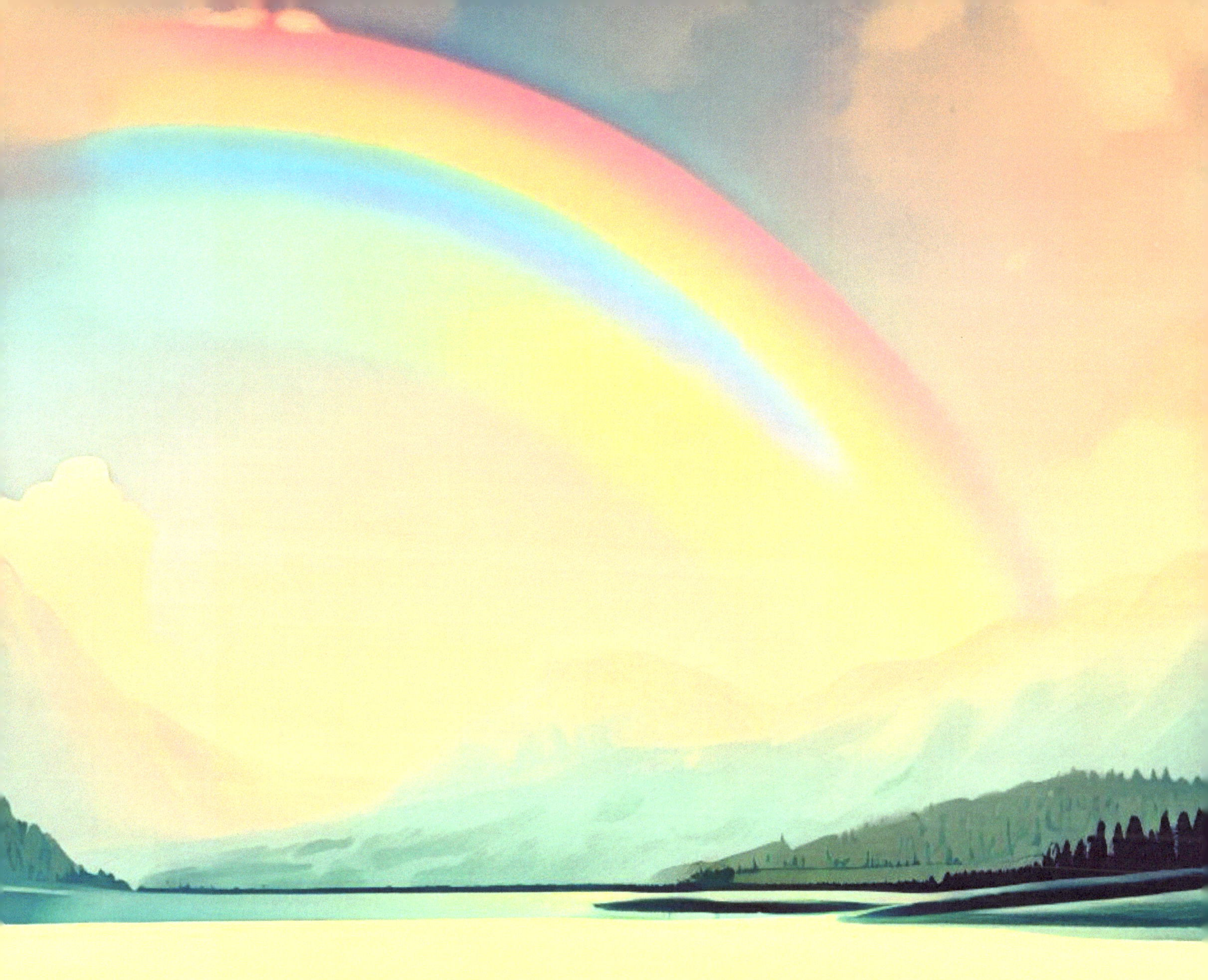
the sky holds up the rainbow
for all its colors to shine.

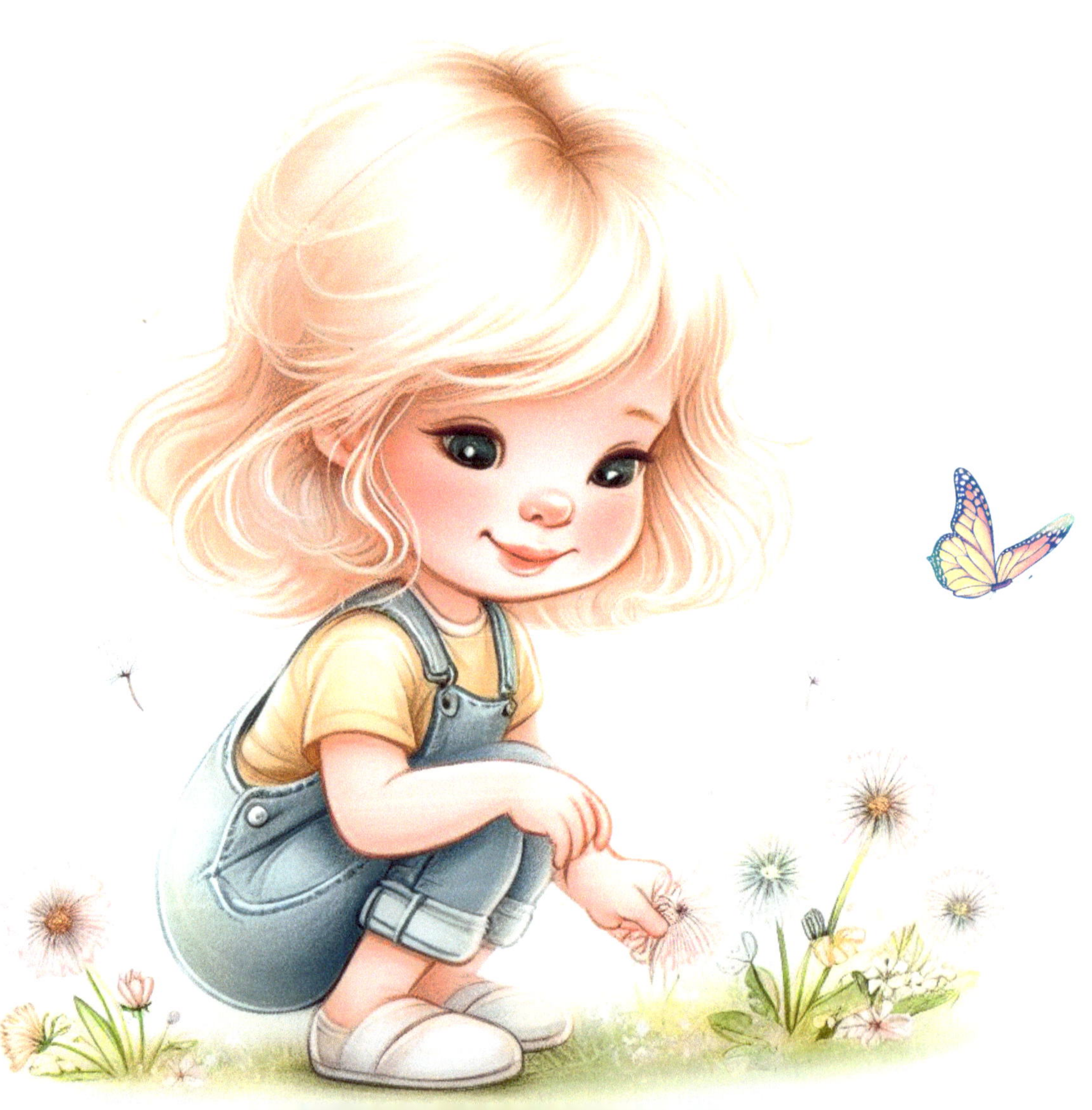

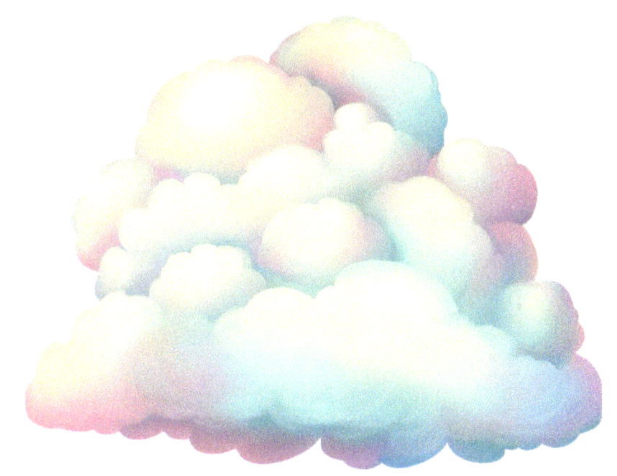

So if ever the world appears somewhat plain,
I hope that you'll pause and look closely again.

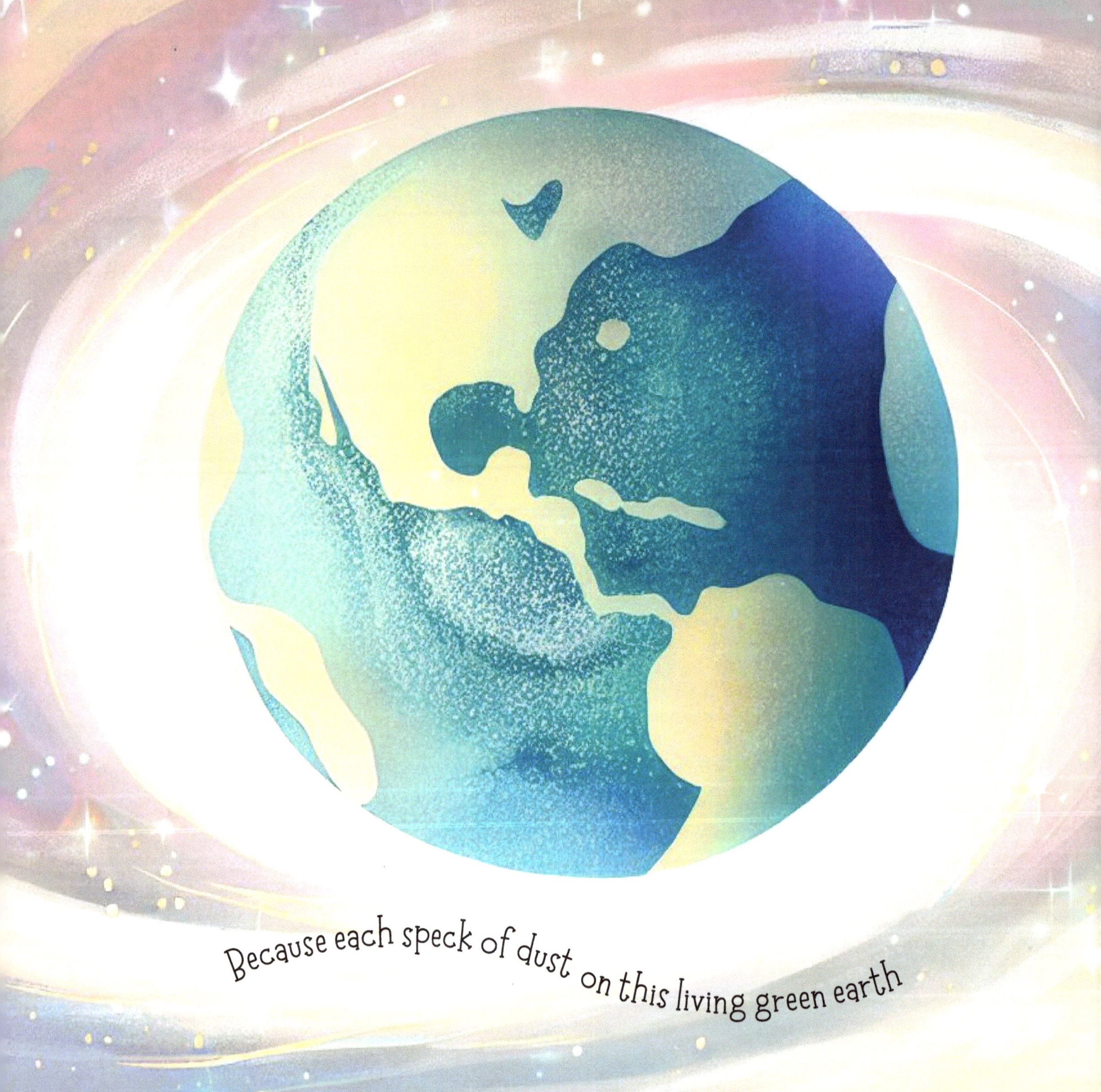
Because each speck of dust on this living green earth

swirled together as one to shape your magical birth.

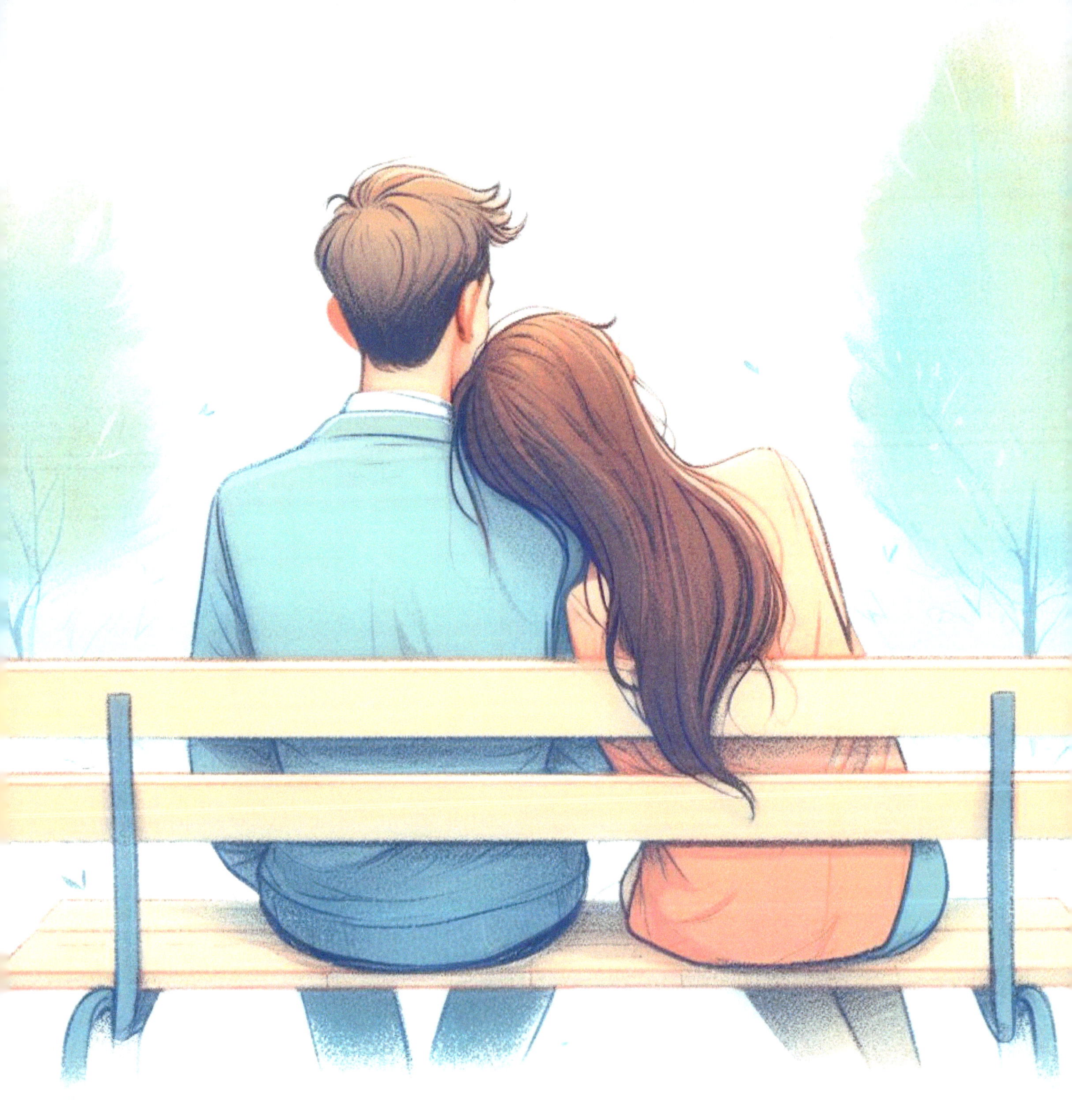

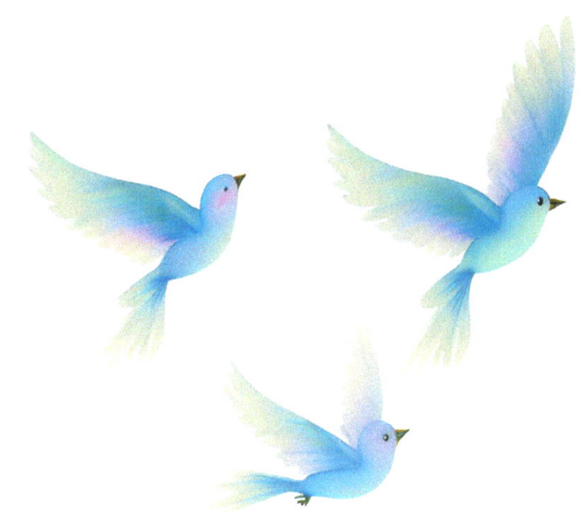

For, when Mommy and Daddy
wished for wonderful you,
we learned that our dream
would take more than just two.

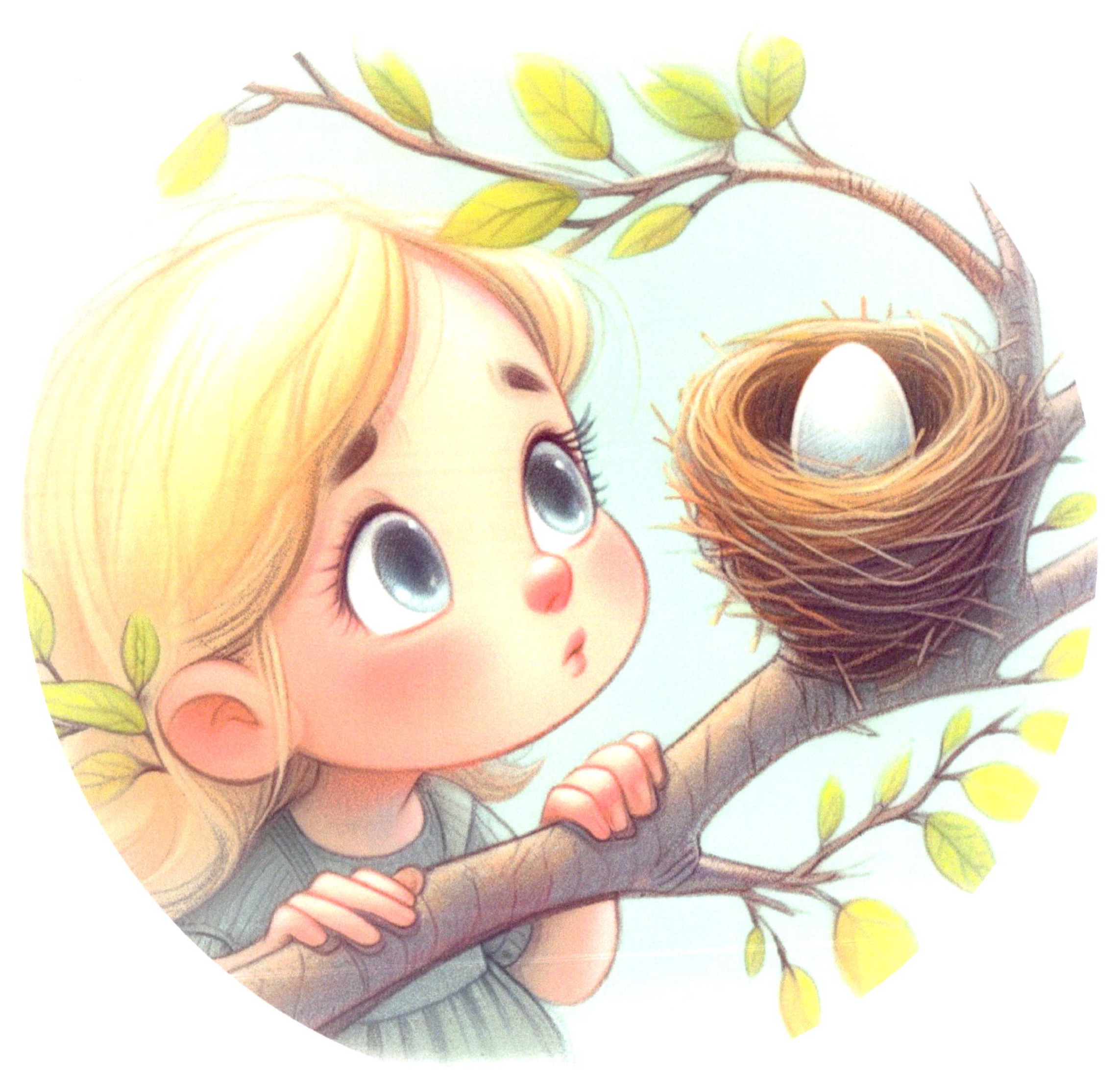

Every new child begins with
one special egg.

But Mommy couldn't use hers,
so to make you instead...

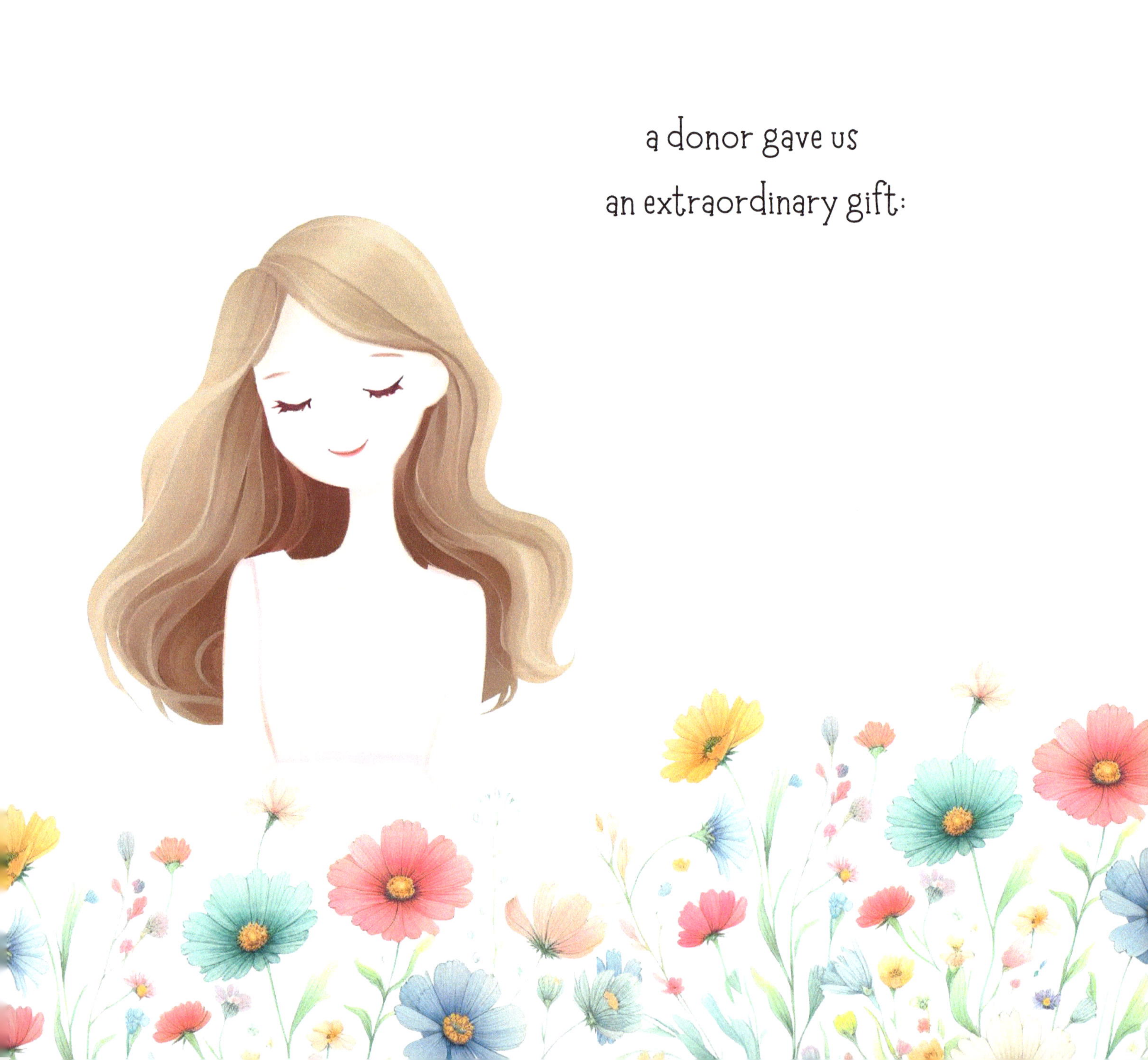

a donor gave us

an extraordinary gift:

one of her eggs, the most

perfect fit.

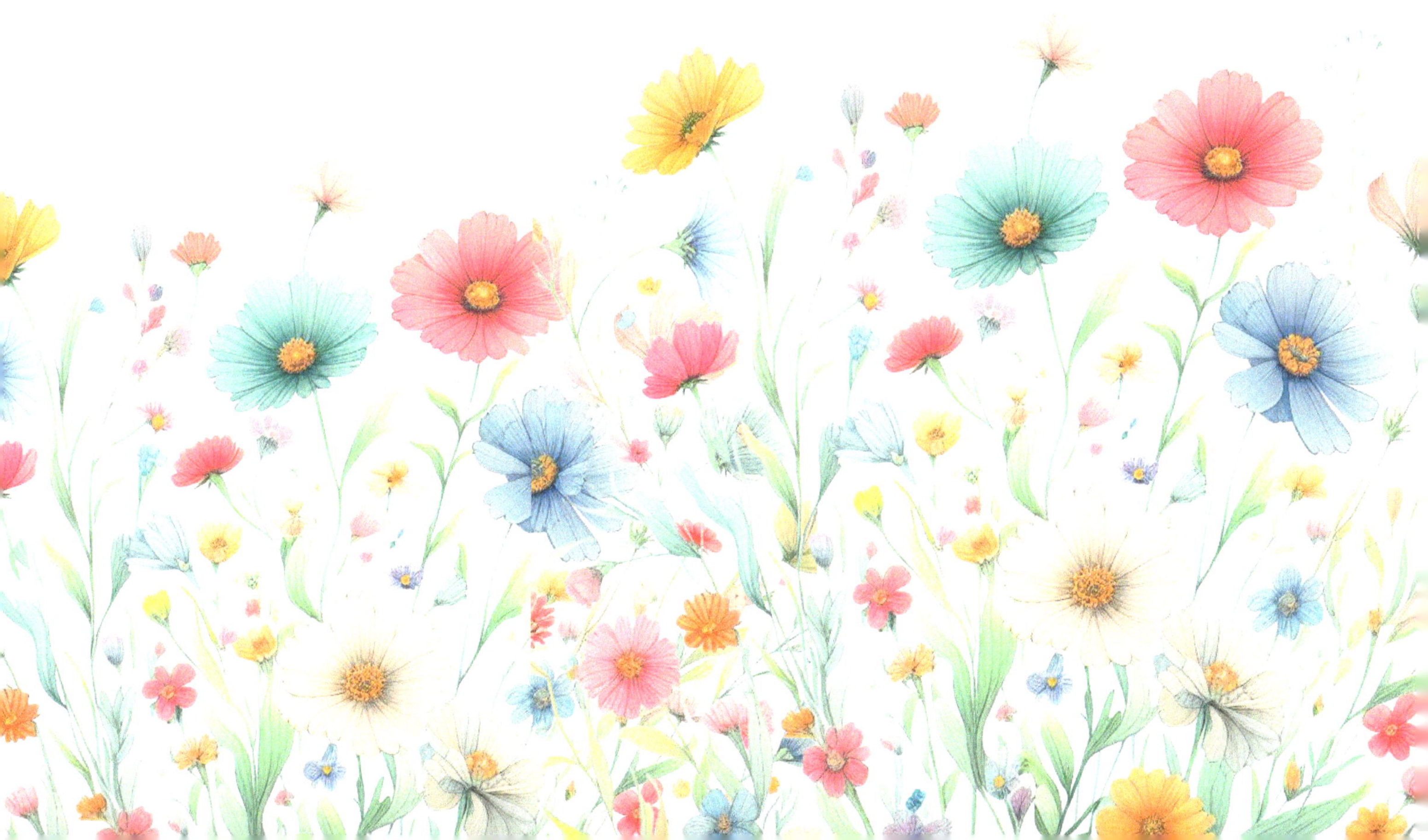

The doctors took care of our new little cell,

uniting it with one from Daddy as well.

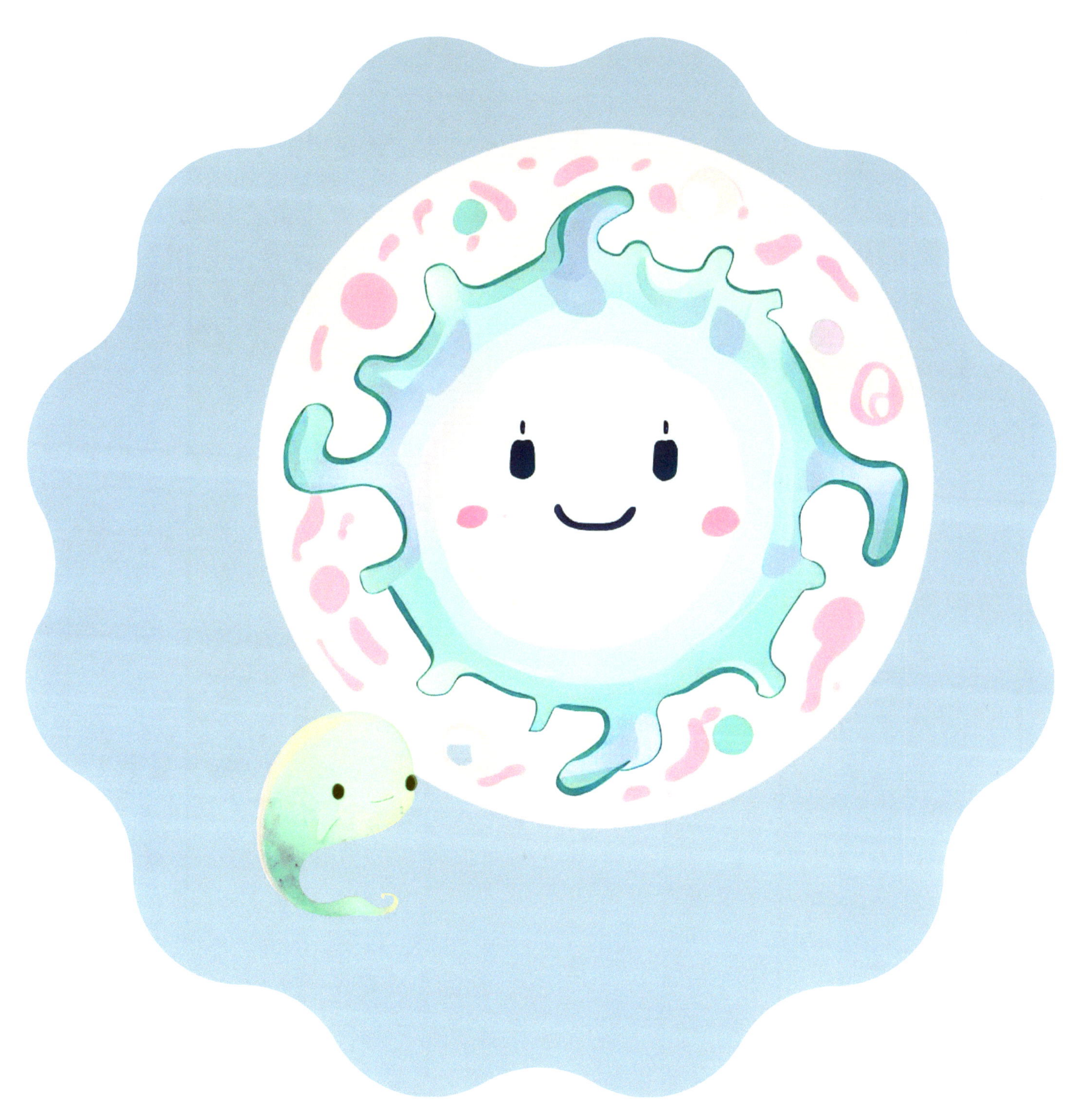

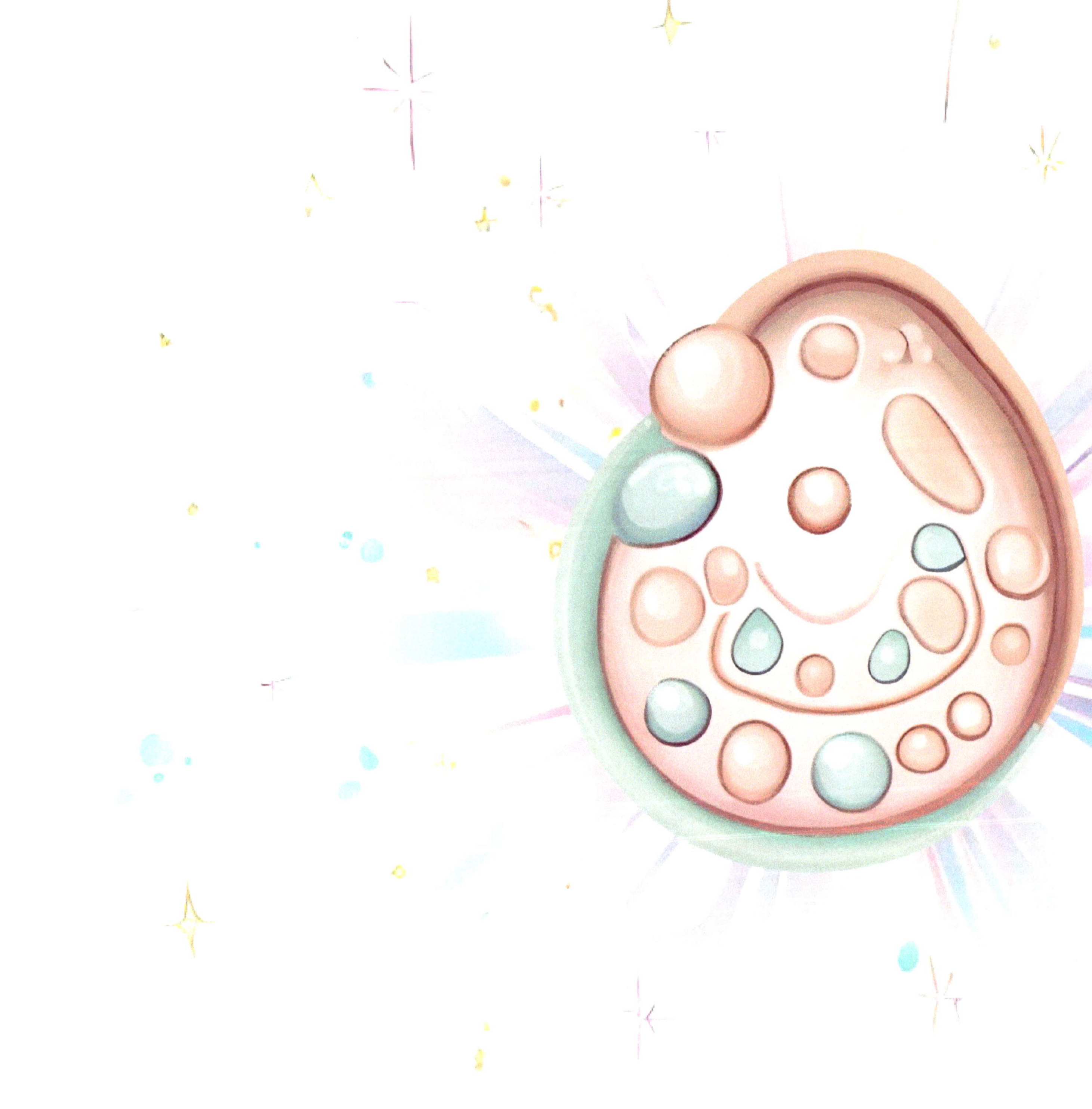

Two joined as one,
and then multiplied
into an embryo
with your beginnings inside.

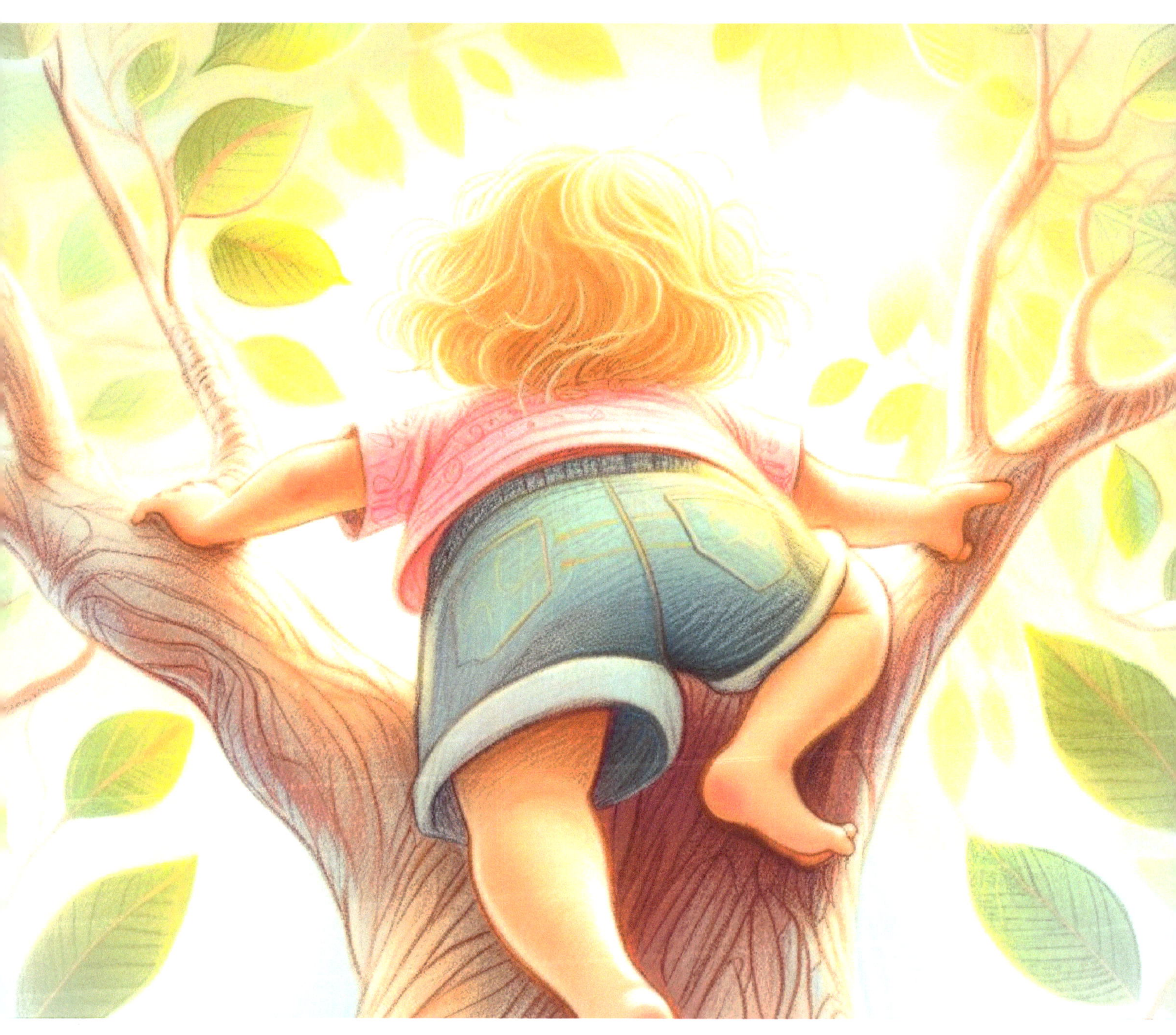

Like a tree's roots
grip the ground down below,
You needed a place
to allow you to grow.

So you lived in Mom's belly — safe, loved, and warm,
while the two of us built an unbreakable bond.

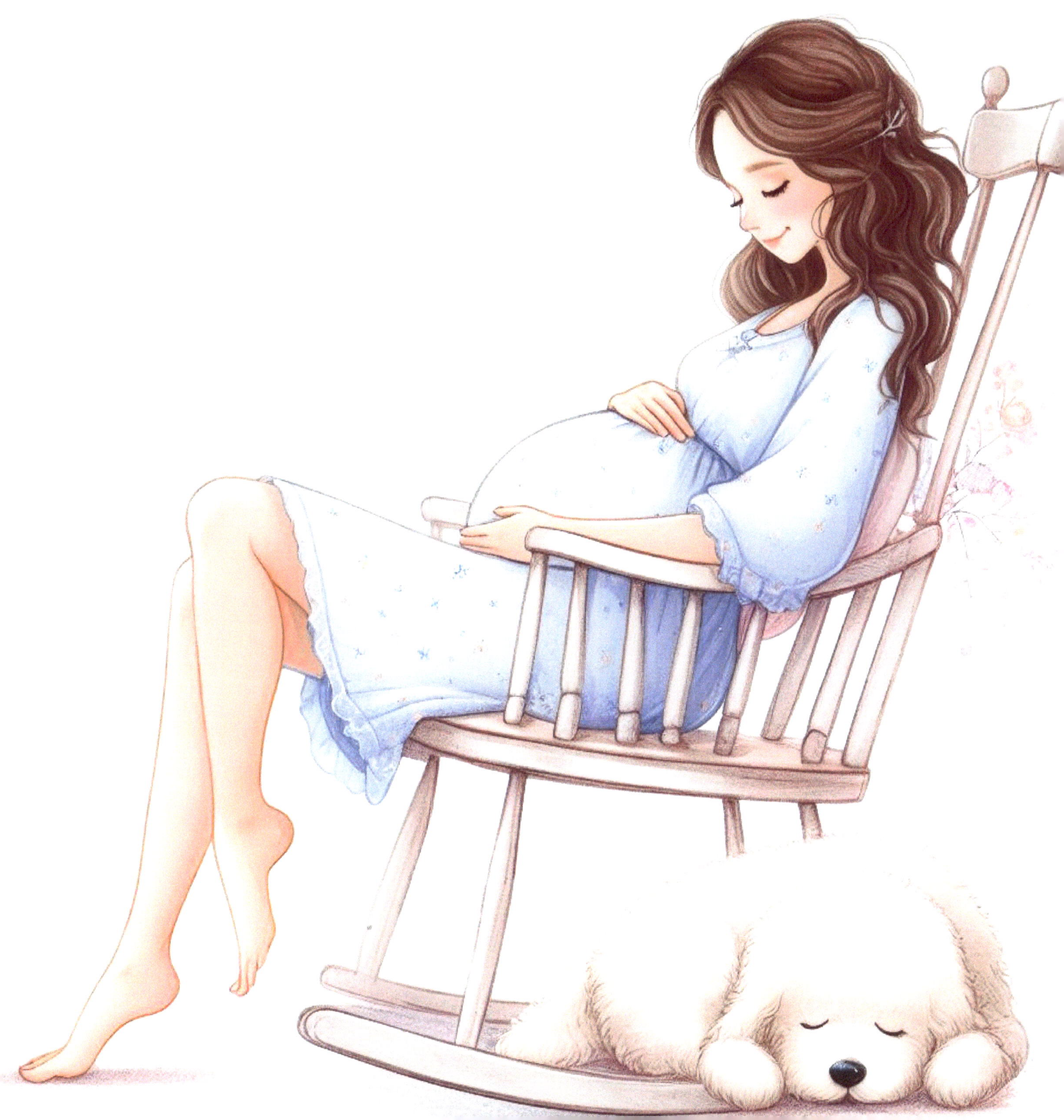

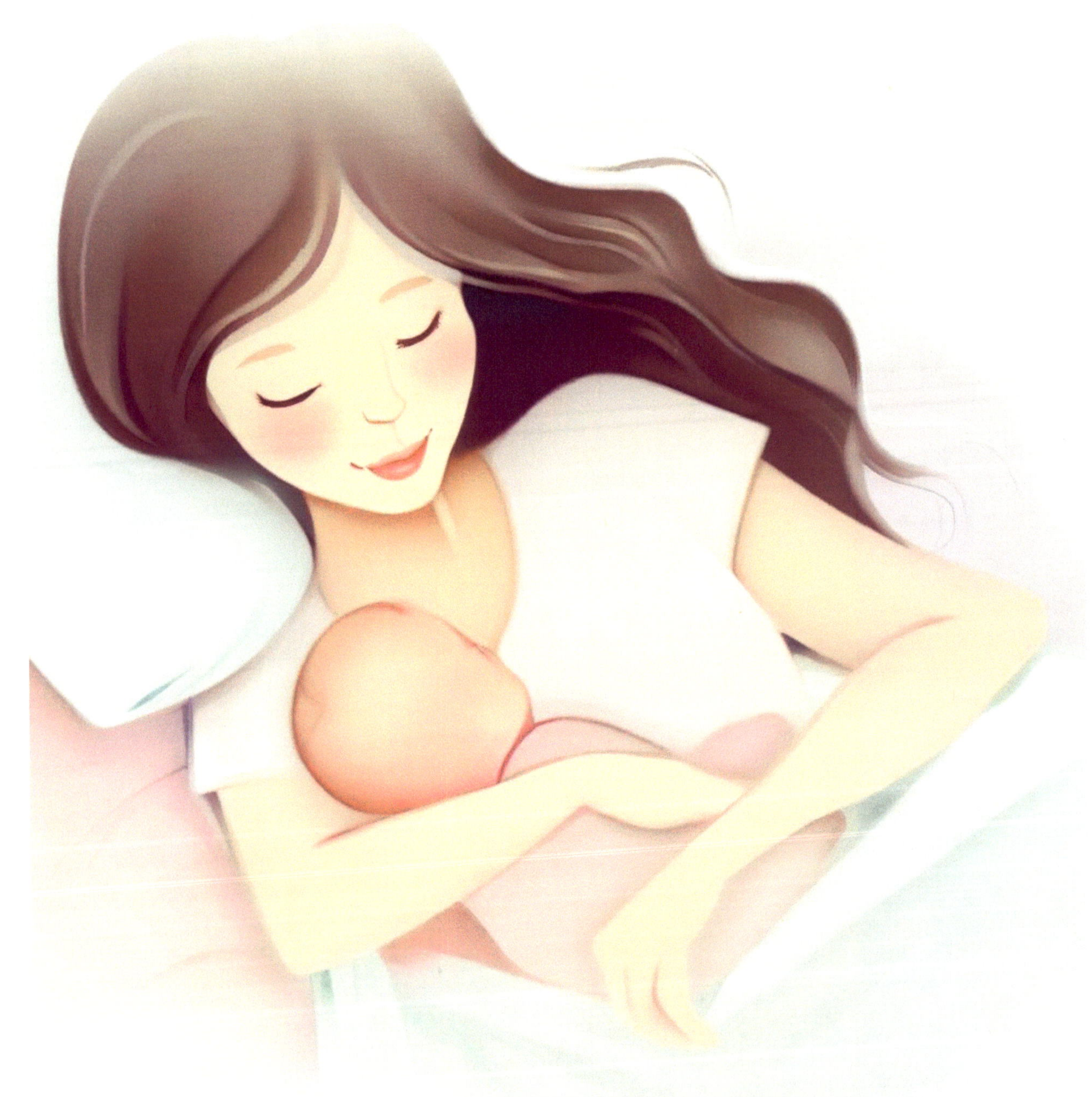

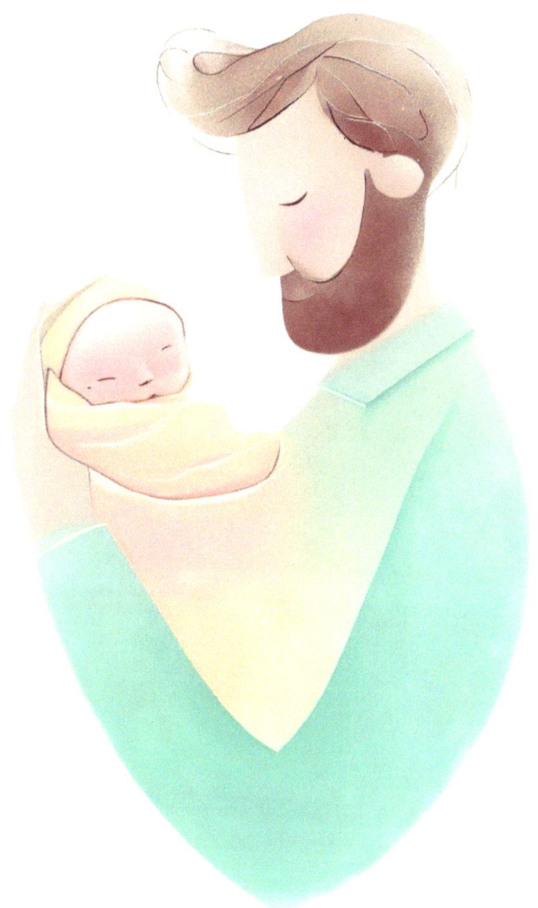

Just as the sand
embraces the tide,
the first time we held you,
our hearts swelled with pride.

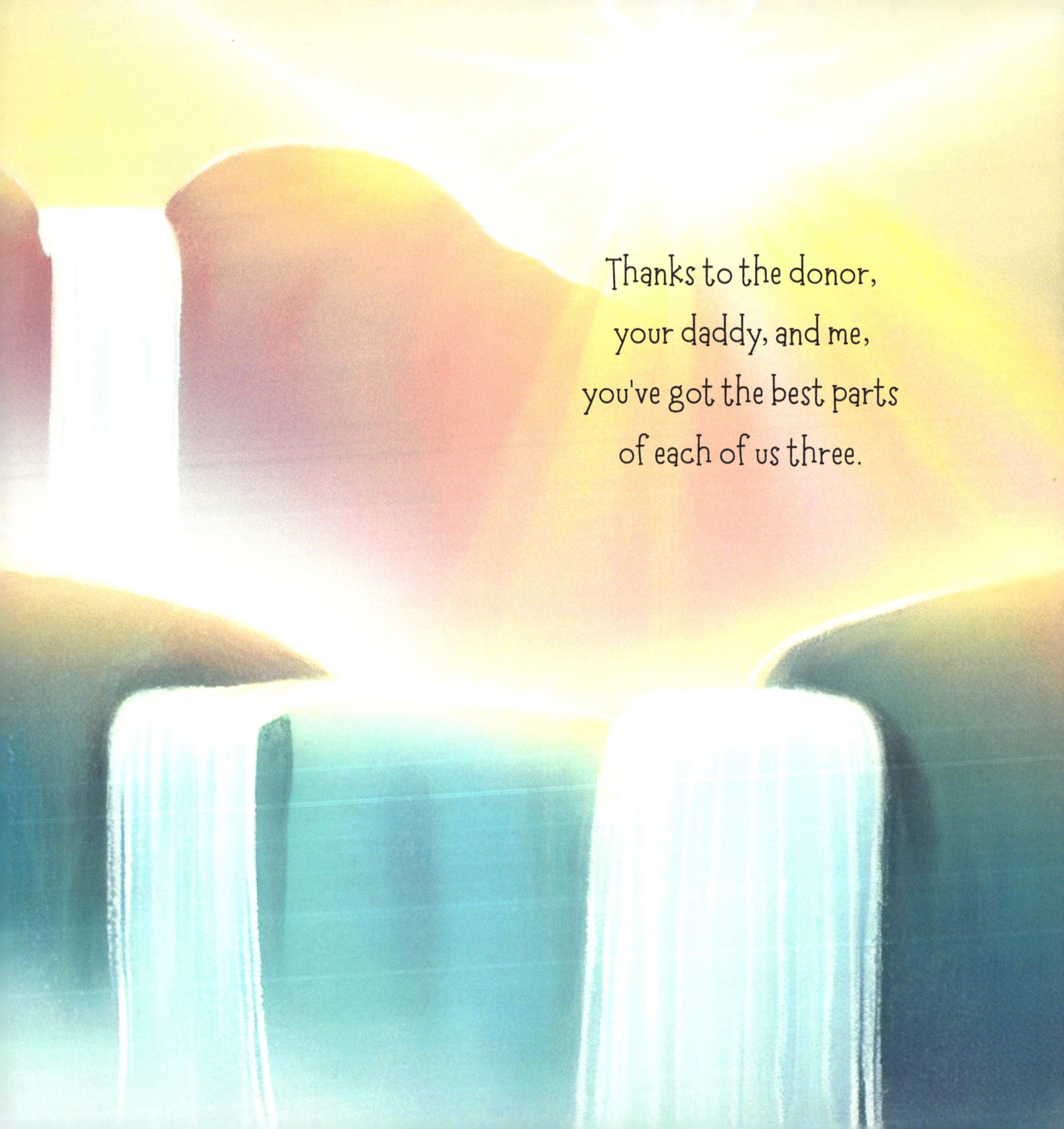

Thanks to the donor,
your daddy, and me,
you've got the best parts
of each of us three.

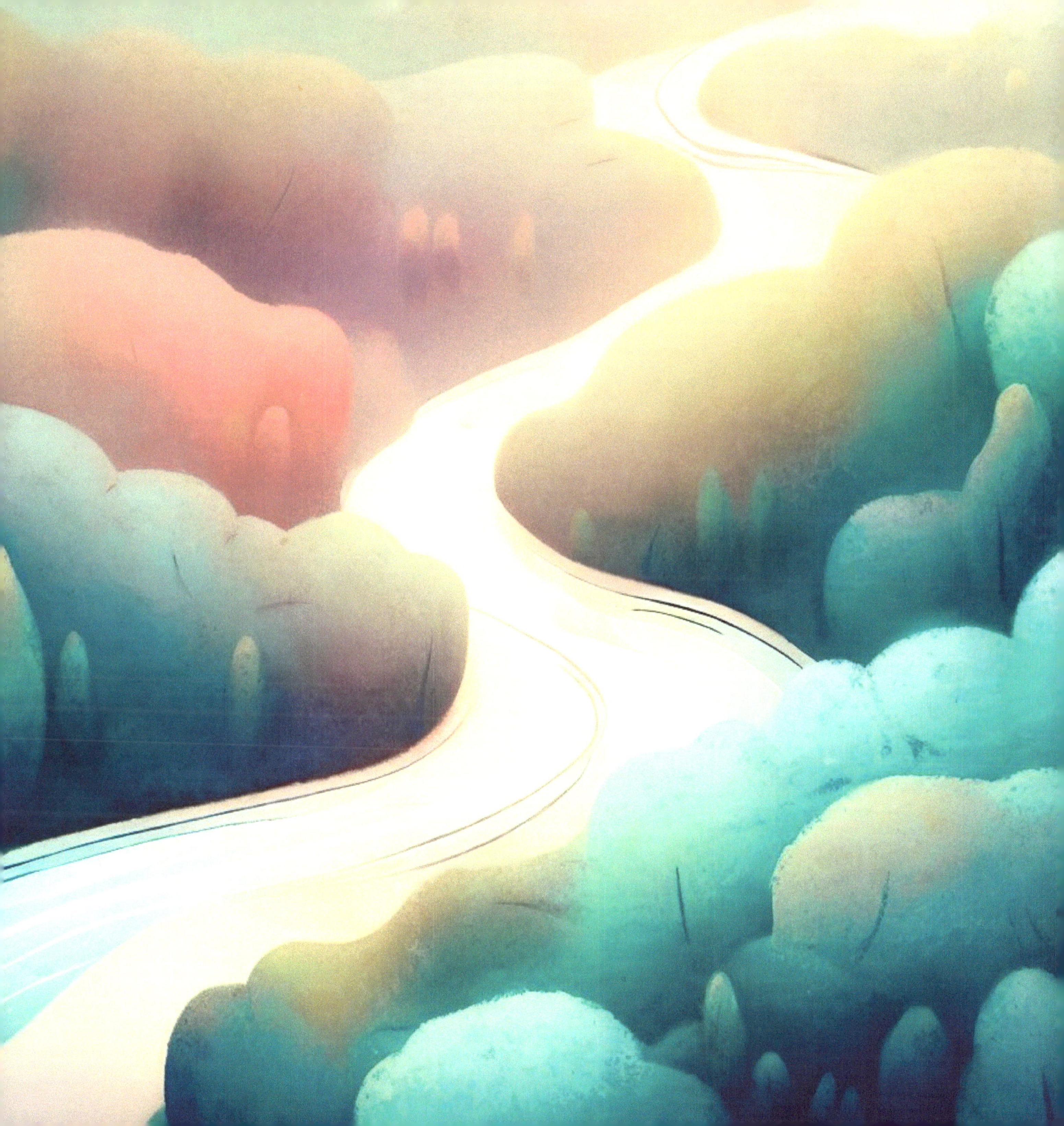

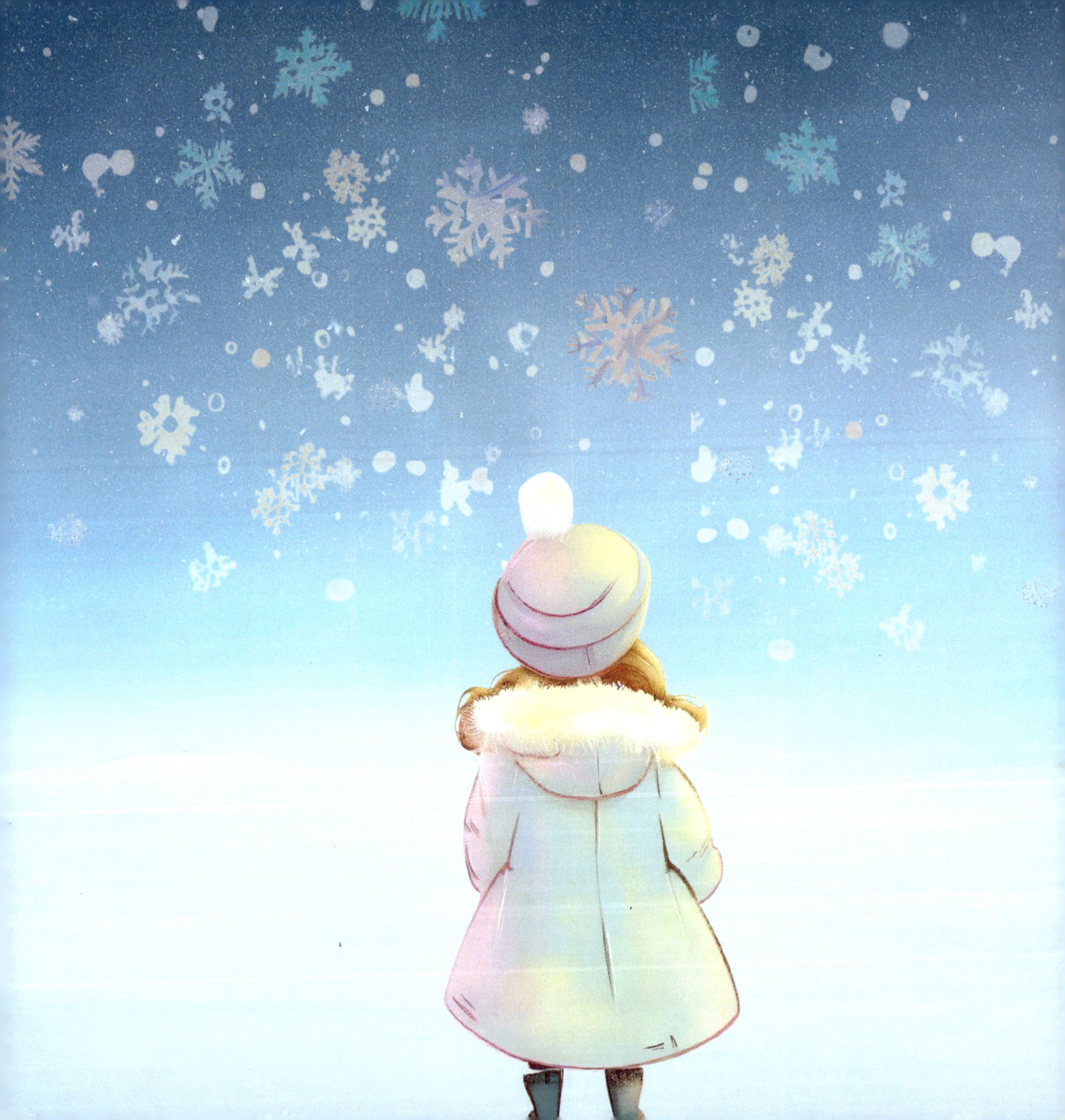

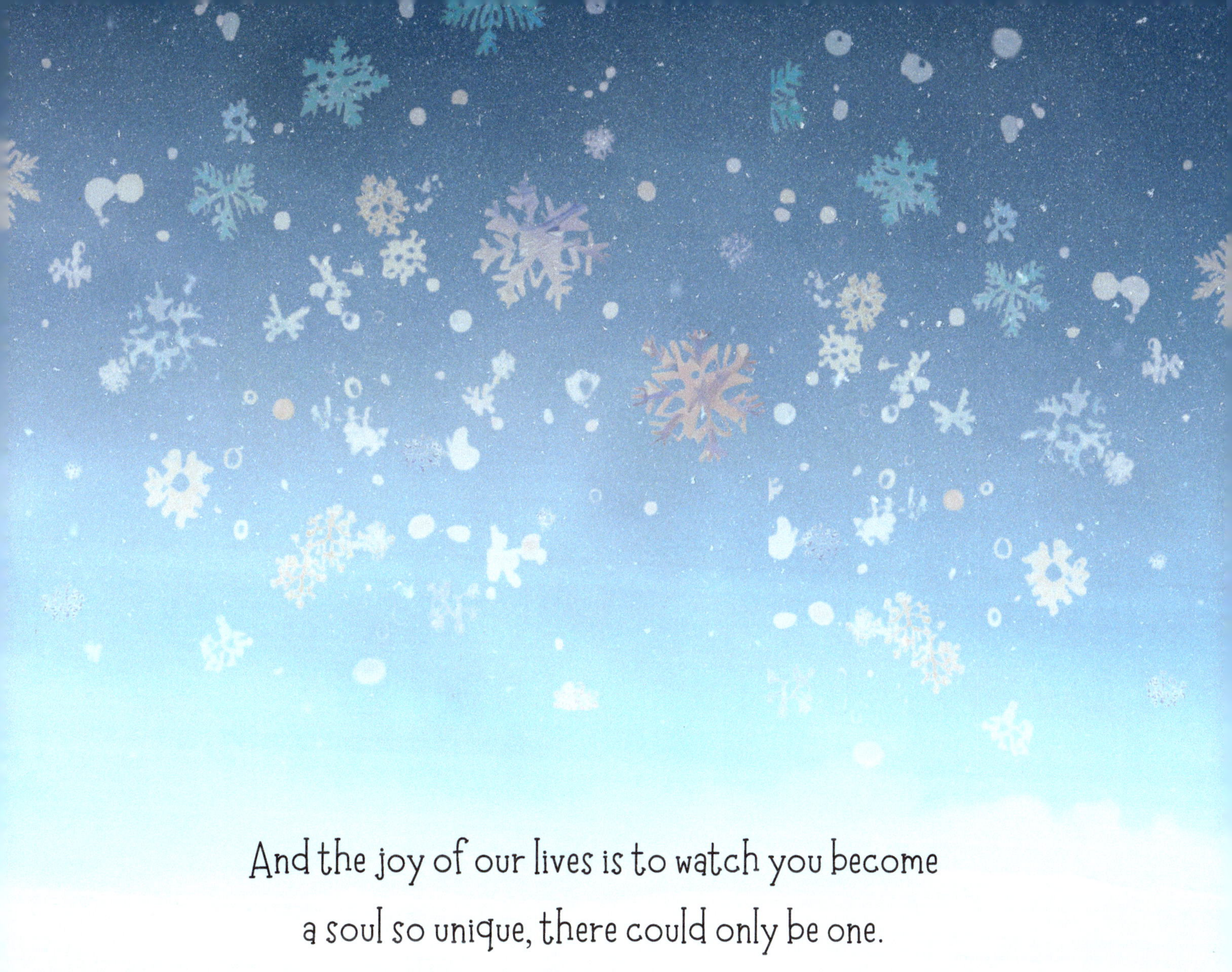

And the joy of our lives is to watch you become
a soul so unique, there could only be one.

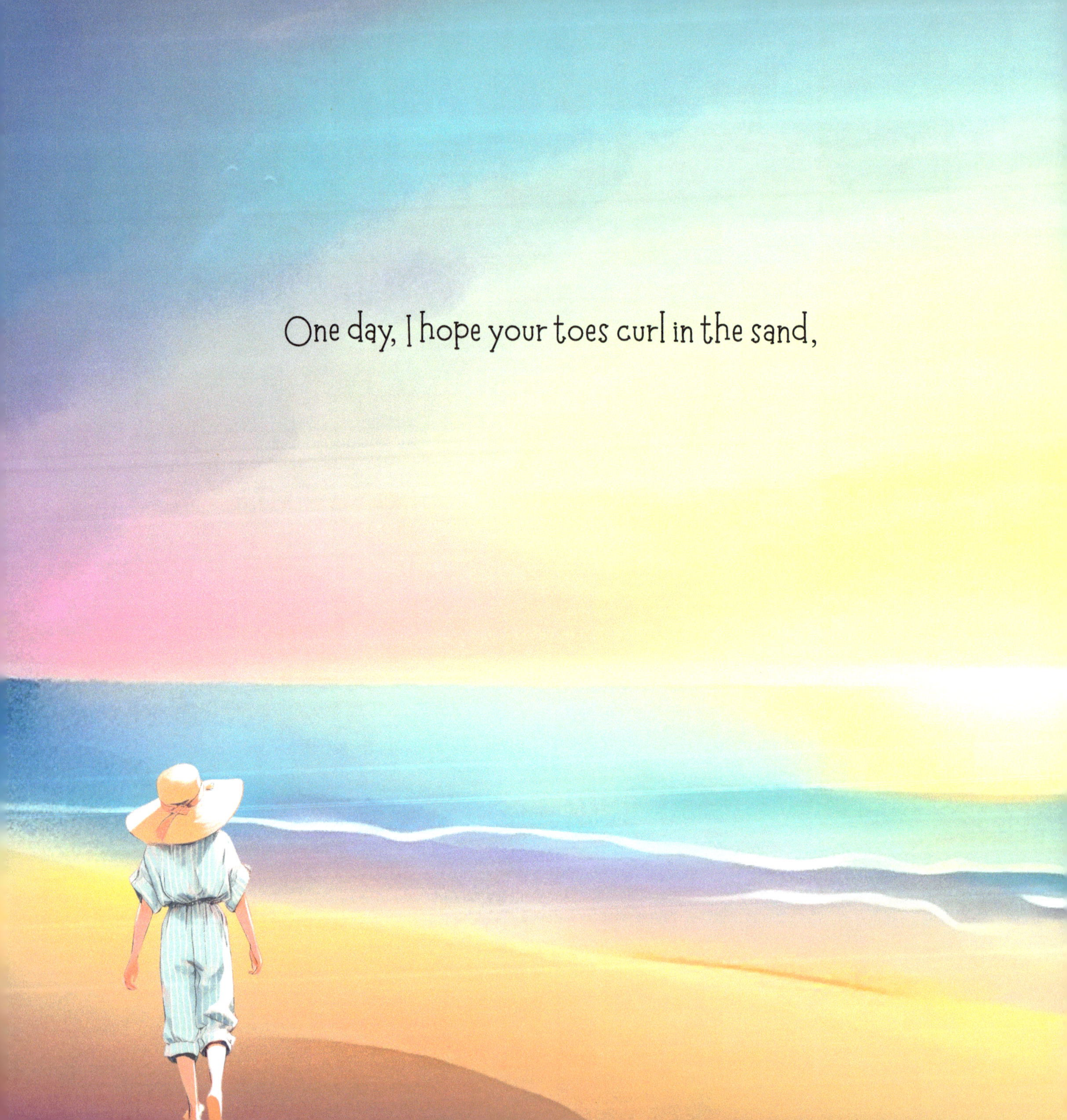
One day, I hope your toes curl in the sand,

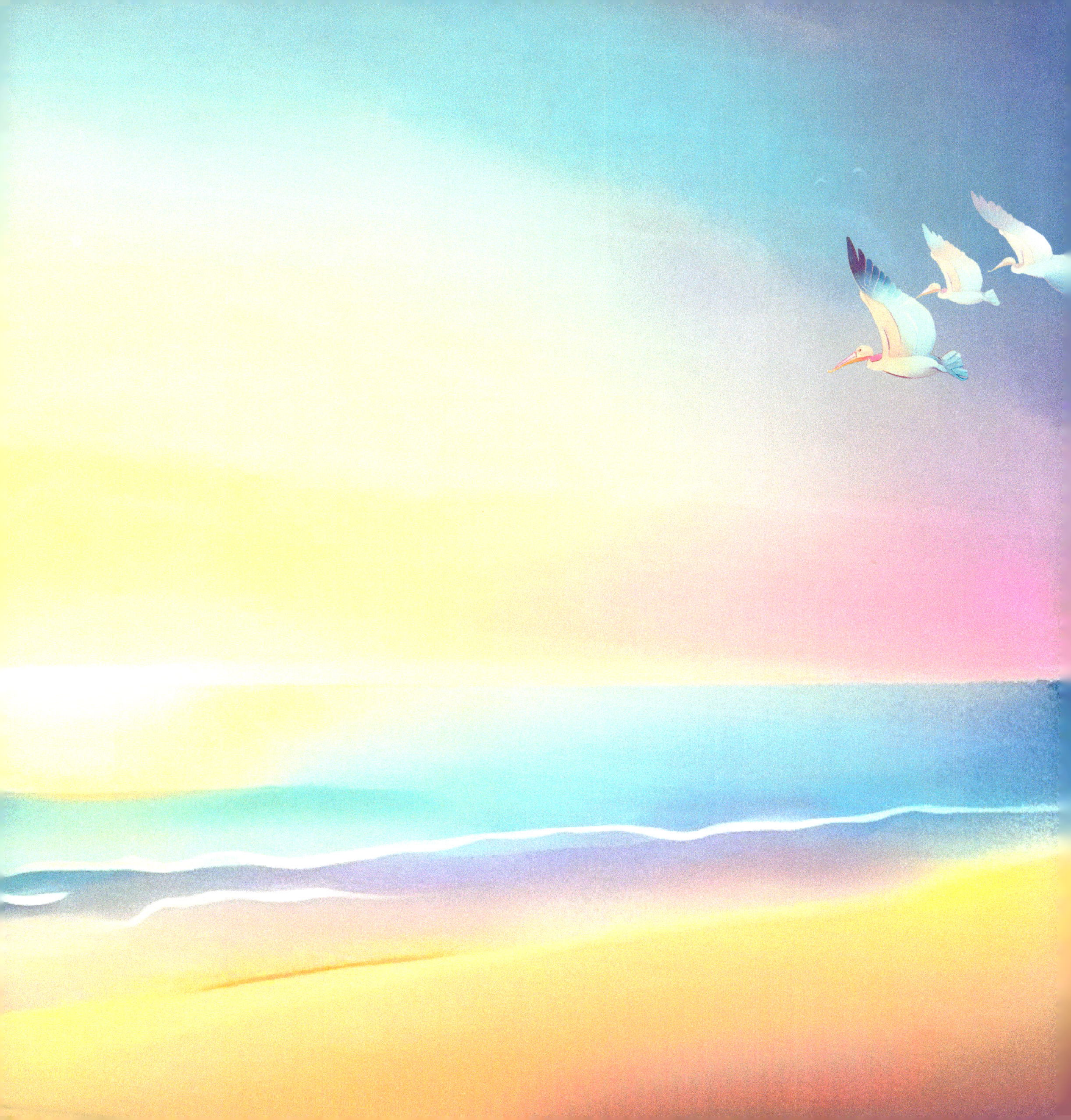

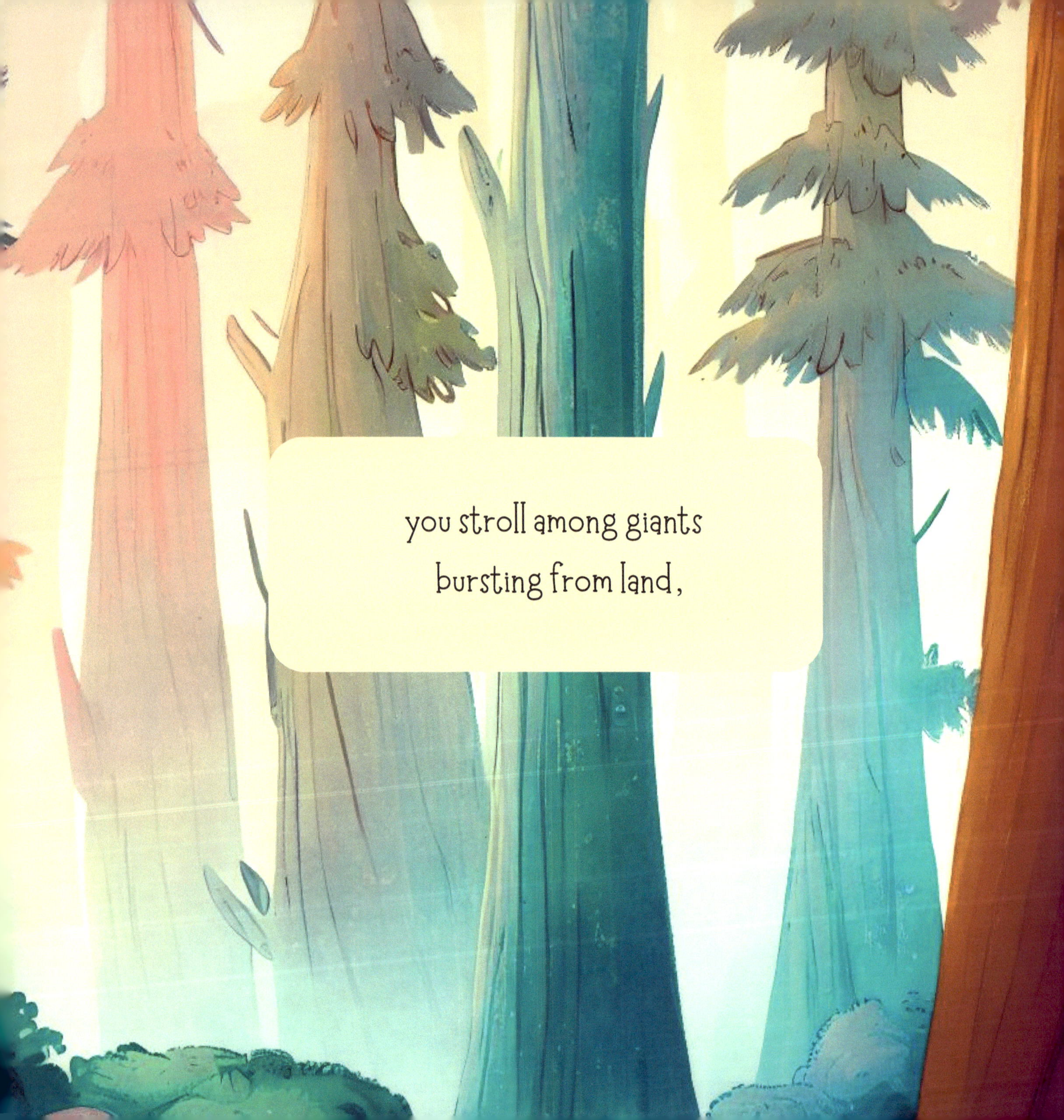

you stroll among giants
bursting from land,

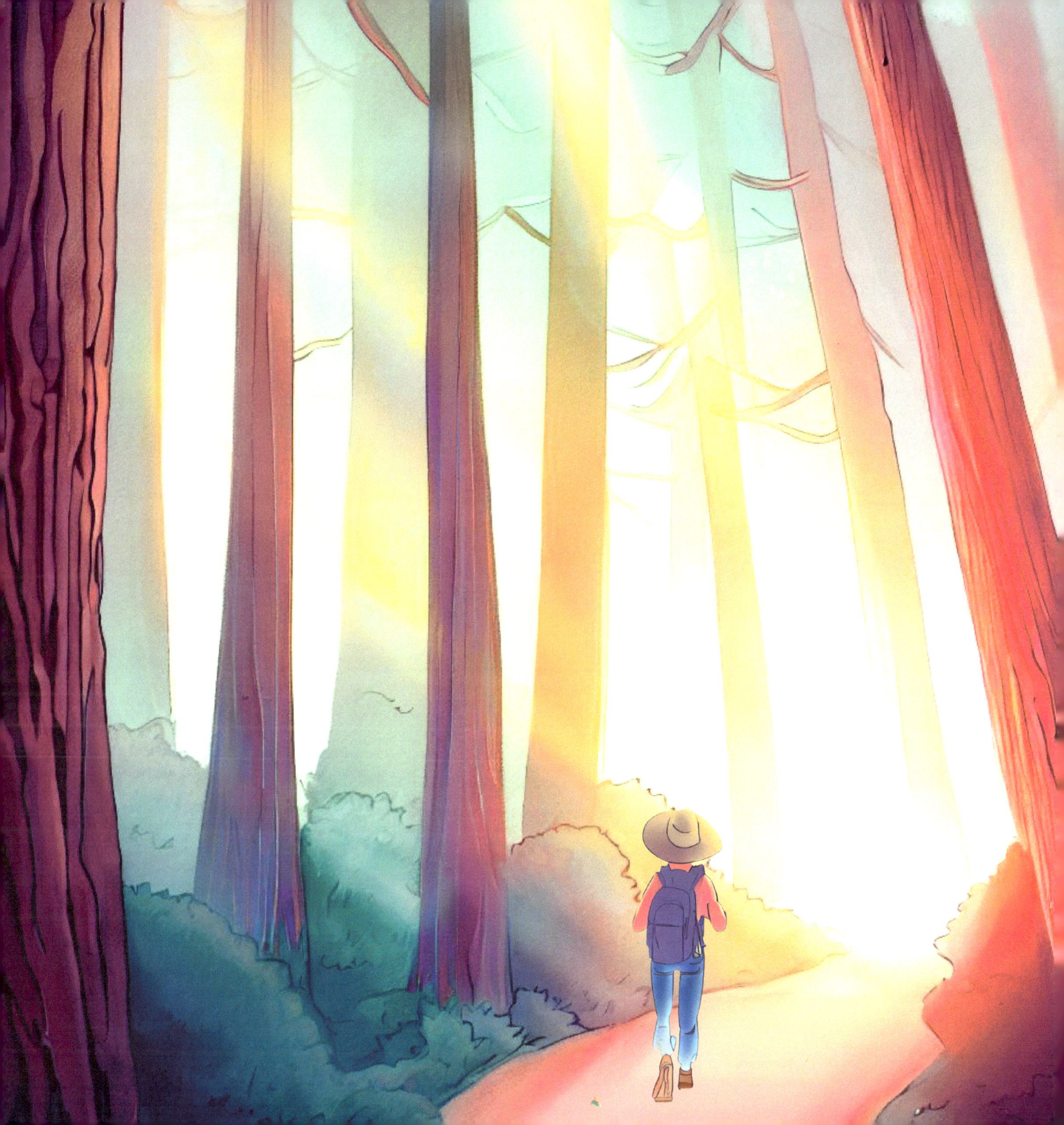

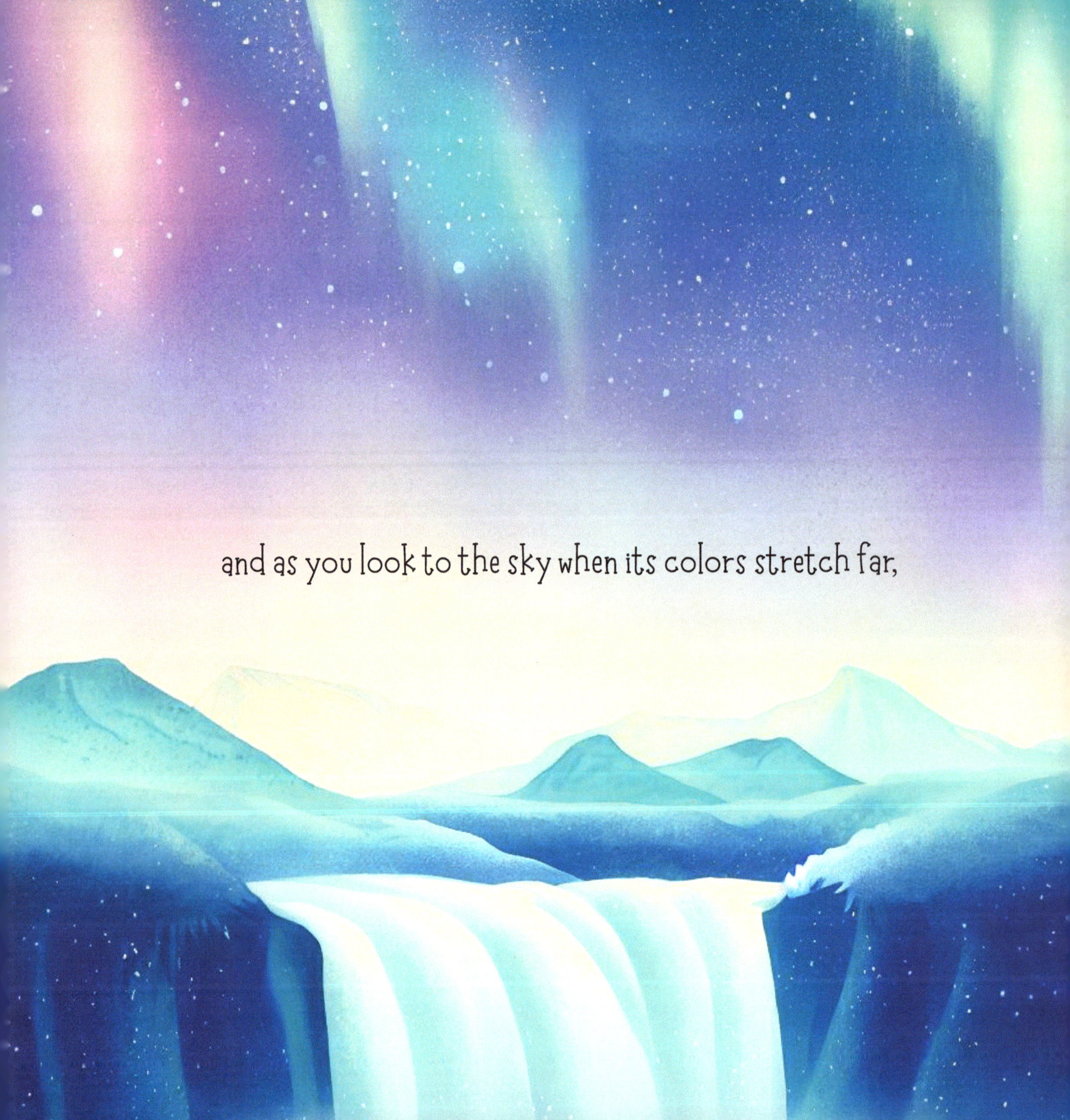
and as you look to the sky when its colors stretch far,

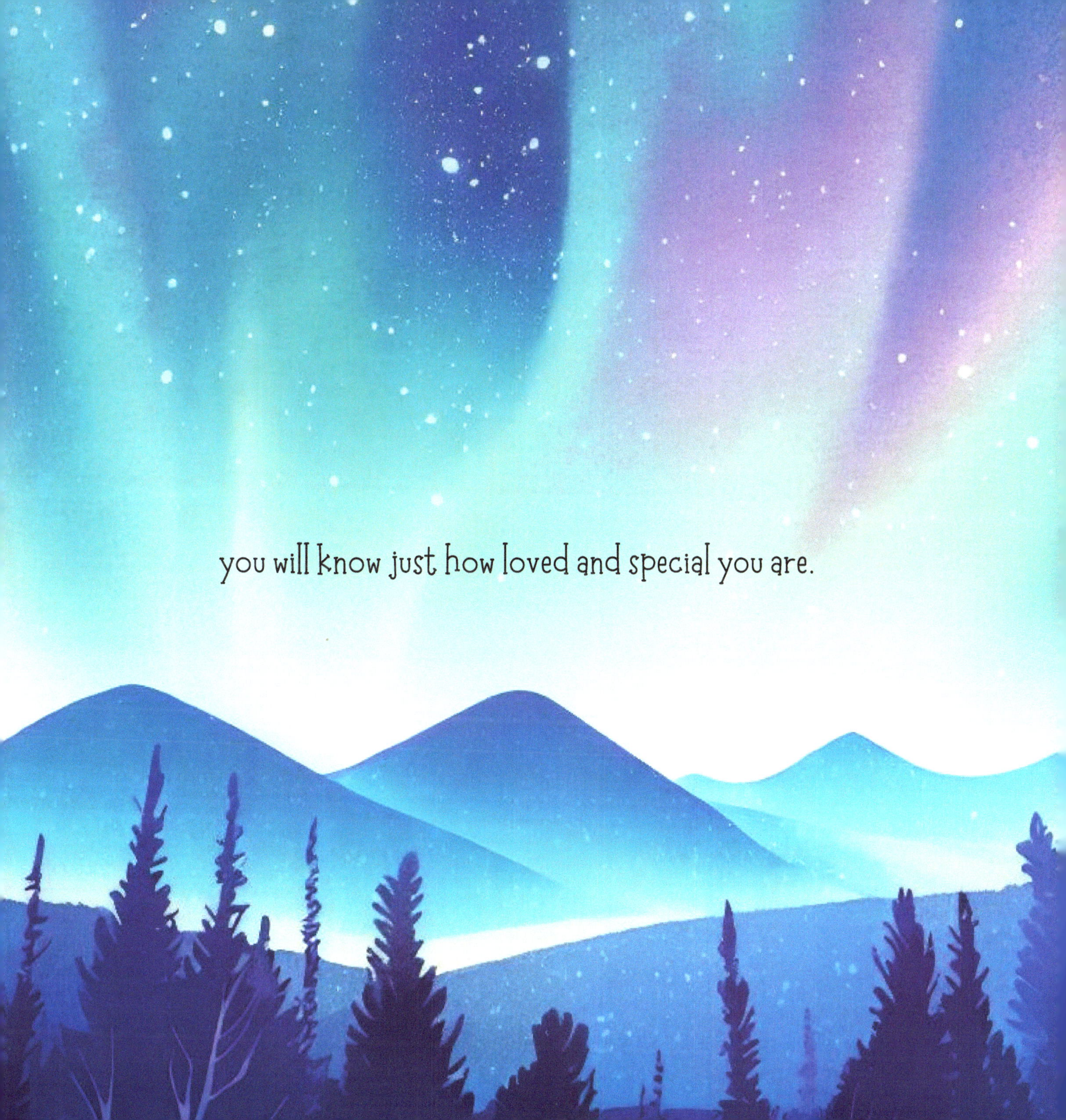
you will know just how loved and special you are.

Written and Illustrated by Nicole Neal
Illustrations created with the
assistance of AI
Independently Published ©2023
ISBN: 9798862213232
First Edition

Contact the author at
authornicoleneal@gmail.com

The author lives in Pennsylvania with her husband.
daughter. and dog. She taught high school
English before becoming a full-time mom and
part-time creator.

9 798862 213232